THE YOGA SUTRAS

OF PATANJALI

Translated with a Preface by
WILLIAM Q. JUDGE

The Yoga Sutras of Patanjali
By Patanjali
Translated with a Preface by William Q. Judge

Print ISBN 13: 978-1-4209-5547-7
eBook ISBN 13: 978-1-4209-5548-4

Cover Image: a detail of "lotus pose yoga chakra symbol, reiki therapy watercolor painting design illustration" by Benjavisa Ruangvaree, Shutterstock Images.

Please visit *www.digireads.com*

CONTENTS

Preface to the First Edition

This edition of Patanjali's Yoga Aphorisms is not put forth as a new translation, nor as a literal rendering into English of the original.

In the year 1885 an edition was printed at Bombay by Mr. Tookeram Tatya, a Fellow of the Theosophical Society, which has been since widely circulated among its members in all parts of the world. But it has been of use only to those who had enough acquaintance with the Indian system of philosophy to enable them to grasp the real meaning of the Aphorisms notwithstanding the great and peculiar obstacles due to the numberless brackets and interpolated sentences with which not only are the Aphorisms crowded, but the so-called explanatory notes as well. For the greater number of readers these difficulties have been an almost insurmountable barrier; and such is the consideration that has led to the preparation of this edition, which attempts to clear up a work that is thought to be of great value to earnest students.

It may be said by some captious critics that liberties have been taken with the text, and if this were emitted as a textual translation the charge would be true. Instead of this being a translation, it is offered as an interpretation, as the thought of Patanjali clothed in our language. No liberties have been taken with the system of the great Sage, but the endeavor has been faithfully to interpret it to Western minds unfamiliar with the Hindu modes of expression, and equally unaccustomed to their philosophy and logic.

About Patanjali's life very little, if anything, can be said. In the *Rudra Jamala*, the *Vrihannan-dikeshwara* and the *Padma-Purana* are some meager statements, more or less legendary, relating to his birth. Illavrita-Varsha is said to have been his birthplace, his mother being Sati the wife of Angira. The tradition runs that upon his birth he made known things past, present and future, showing the intellect and penetration of a sage while yet an infant. He is said to have married one Lolupa, whom he found in the hollow of a tree on the north of Sumeru, and thereafter to have lived to a great age. On one occasion, being insulted by the inhabitants of Bhotabhandra while he was engaged in religious austerities, he reduced them to ashes by fire from his mouth.

That these accounts are legendary and symbolical can be easily seen. Illavrita-Varsha is no part of India, but is some celestial abode. The name of India proper is Bharata Varsha. "In it and nowhere else do the four ages or Yugas—Krita, Treta, Dwapara and Kali—exist. Here devotees perform austerities and priests sacrifice. In this respect Bharata is the most excellent division; for this is the land of works, while the others are places of enjoyment." In the Bhagavat-Purana it is said: "Of the Varshas, Bharata alone is the land of works; the other eight (including Illavrita-Varsha) are places where the celestials enjoy the remaining rewards of their works." As Bharata-Varsha is a division of Jambudwipa, and known as India, and the other Varshas are for celestials, it follows that the account of Patanjali's birthplace cannot be relied upon in a material sense. It may be the ancient method of showing how great sages now and then descend from other spheres to aid and benefit man. But there is also another Patanjali mentioned in the Indian books. He was born in India at Gonarda, in the east, and from there be went to reside temporarily in Kashmir. Prof. Goldstücker has concluded that this later Patanjali wrote about 140 B.C. His writings were commentaries upon the great grammarian Panini, and it is in respect to the Sanskrit language that he is regarded as an authority. He must not be confounded with our Patanjali; of the latter all that we have is the Philosophy set forth in the Aphorisms.

In regard to the systems of Yoga, we cannot do better than to quote some introductory remarks made by Col. H. S. Olcott, President of the Theosophical Society, in the Bombay edition of these Aphorisms, in August, 1885. He said:

"The Yoga system is divided into two principal parts—Hatha and Raja Yoga. There are many minor divisions which can be brought under either of these heads. Hatha Yoga was promoted and practiced by Matsendra Nath and Goraksh Nath and their followers, and by many sects of ascetics in this country (India). This system deals principally with the physiological part of man with a view to establish his health and train his will. The processes prescribed to arrive at this end are so difficult that only a few resolute souls go through all the stages of its practice, while many have failed and died in the attempt. It is therefore strongly denounced by all the philosophers. The most illustrious Sankarâchârya has remarked in his treatise called Aparokshanubhuti that 'the system of Hatha Yoga was intended for those whose worldly desires are not pacified or uprooted.' He has strongly spoken elsewhere against this practice.

"On the other hand, the Raja Yogis try to control the mind itself by following the rules laid down by the greatest of adepts."

Patanjali's rules compel the student not only to acquire a right knowledge of what is and what is not real, but also to practice all virtues, and while results in the way of psychic development are not so immediately seen as in the case of the successful practitioner of Hatha Yoga, it is infinitely safer and is certainly spiritual, which Hatha Yoga is not. In Patanjali's Aphorisms there is some slight allusion to the practices of Hatha Yoga, such as "postures," each of which is more difficult than those preceding, and "retention of the breath," but he distinctly says that mortification and other practices are either for the purpose of extenuating certain mental afflictions or for the more easy attainment of concentration of mind.

In Hatha Yoga practice, on the contrary, the result is psychic development at the delay or expense of the spiritual nature. These last named practices and results may allure the Western student, but from our knowledge of inherent racial difficulties there is not much fear that many will persist in them.

This book is meant for sincere students, and especially for those who have some glimmering of what Krishna meant, when in *Bhagavad-Gita* he said, that after a while spiritual knowledge grows up within and illuminates with its rays all subjects and objects. Students of the mere forms of Sanskrit who look for new renderings or laborious attempts at altering the meaning of words and sentences will find nothing between these covers.

It should be ever borne in mind that Patanjali had no need to assert or enforce the doctrine of reincarnation. That is assumed all through the Aphorisms. That it could be doubted, or need any restatement, never occurred to him, and by us it is alluded to, not because we have the smallest doubt of its truth, but only because we see about us those who never heard of such a doctrine, who, educated under the frightful dogmas of Christian priestcraft, imagine that upon quitting this life they will enjoy heaven or be damned eternally, and who not once pause to ask where was their soul before it came into the present body.

Without Reincarnation Patanjali's Aphorisms are worthless. Take No. 18, Book III, which declares that the ascetic can know what were his previous incarnations with all their circumstances; or No. 13, Book II, that while there is a root of works there is fructification in rank and years and experience. Both of these infer reincarnation. In Aphorism 8, Book IV, reincarnation is a necessity. The manifestation, in any incarnation, of the effects of mental deposits made in previous lives, is declared to ensue upon the obtaining of just the kind of bodily and mental frame, constitution and environment as will bring them out. Where were these deposits received if not in preceding lives on earth—or even if on other planets, it is still reincarnation. And so on all through the Aphorisms this law is tacitly admitted.

In order to understand the system expounded in this book it is also necessary to admit the existence of soul, and the comparative unimportance of the body in which it dwells. For Patanjali holds that Nature exists for the soul's sake, taking it for granted that the student believes in the existence of soul. Hence he does not go into proof of that which in his day was admitted on every hand. And, as he lays down that the real experiencer and knower is the soul and not the mind, it follows that the Mind, designated either as "internal organ," or "thinking principle," while higher and more subtle than the body, is yet only an instrument used by the Soul in gaining experience, just in the same way as an astronomer uses his telescope for acquiring information respecting the heavens. But the Mind is a most important factor in the pursuit of concentration; one indeed without which concentration cannot be obtained, and therefore we see in the first book that to this subject Patanjali devotes attention. He shows that the mind is, as he terms it, "modified" by any object or subject brought before it, or to which it is directed. This may be well illustrated by quoting a passage from the commentator, who says: "The internal organ is there"—in the *Vedanta Paribhasha*—"compared to water in respect of its readiness to adapt itself to the form of whatever mold it may enter. 'As the waters of a reservoir, having issued from an aperture, having entered by a channel the basins, become four-cornered or otherwise shaped, just like them; so the manifesting internal organ having gone through the sight, or other channel, to where there is one object, for instance a jar, becomes modified by the form of the jar or other object. It is this altered state of the internal organ—or mind—that is called its modification.'" While the internal organ thus molds itself upon the object it at the same time reflects it and its properties to the soul. The channels by which the mind is held to go out to an object or subject, are the organs of sight, touch, taste, hearing, and so on. Hence by means of hearing it shapes itself into the form of the idea which may be given in speech, or by means of the eye in reading, it is molded into the form of that which is read; again, sensations such as heat and cold modify it directly and indirectly by association and by recollection, and similarly in the ease of all senses and sensations.

It is further held that this internal organ, while having an innate disposition to assume some modification or other depending upon constantly recurring objects—whether directly present or only such as arise from the power of reproducing thoughts, whether by association or otherwise, may be controlled and stilled into a state of absolute calmness. This is what he means by "hindering the modifications." And just here it is seen that the theory of the soul's being the real experiencer and knower is necessary. For if we are but mind, or slaves of mind, we never can attain real knowledge because the incessant panorama of objects eternally modifies that mind which is uncontrolled by the soul, always preventing real knowledge from being acquired. But as the Soul is held to be superior to Mind, it has the power to grasp and hold the latter if we but use the will to aid it in the work, and then only the real end and purpose of mind is brought about.

These propositions imply that the will is not wholly dependent on the mind, but is separable from it; and, further, that knowledge exists as an abstraction. The will and mind are only servants for the soul's use, but so long as we are wrapped up in material life and do not admit that the real knower and only experiencer is the soul, just so long do these servants remain usurpers of the soul's sovereignty. Hence it is stated in old Hindu works, that "the Soul is the friend of Self and also its enemy; and, that a man should raise the self by the self."

In other words there is a constant struggle between the lower and the Higher Self, in which the illusions of matter always wage war against the Soul, tending ever to draw downward the inner principles which, lying midway between the upper and the lower, are capable of reaching either salvation or damnation.

There is no reference in the Aphorisms to the will. It seems to be inferred, either as well understood and admitted, or as being one of the powers of soul itself and not to be discussed. Many old Hindu writers hold, and we incline to the same view, that Will is a spiritual power, function or attribute constantly present in every portion of the Universe. It is a colorless power, to which no quality of goodness or badness is to be assigned, but which may be used in whatever way man pleases. When considered as that which in ordinary life is called "will," we see its operation only in connection with the material body and mind guided by desire; looked at in respect to the hold by man upon life it is more recondite, because its operation is beyond the ken of the mind; analyzed as connected with reincarnation of man or with the persistence of the manifested universe throughout a Manvantara, it is found to be still more removed from our comprehension and vast in its scope.

In ordinary life it is not man's servant, but, being then guided solely by desire, it makes man a slave to his desires. Hence the old cabalistic maxim, "Behind Will stands Desire." The desires always drawing the man hither and thither, cause him to commit such actions and have such thoughts as form the cause and mold for numerous reincarnations, enslaving him to a destiny against which he rebels, and that constantly destroys and re-creates his mortal body. It is an error to say of those who are known as strong-willed men, that their wills are wholly their servants, for they are so bound in desire that it, being strong, moves the will into action for the consummation of wished for ends. Every day we see good and evil men prevailing in their several spheres. To say that in one there is good, and in the other evil will is manifestly erroneous and due to mistaking will, the instrument or force, for desire that sets it in motion toward a good or bad purpose. But Patanjali and his school well knew that the secret of directing the will with ten times the ordinary force might be discovered if they outlined the method, and then bad men whose desires were strong and conscience wanting, would use it with impunity against their fellows; or that even sincere students might be carried away from spirituality when dazzled by the wonderful results flowing from a training of the will alone. Patanjali is silent upon the subject for this reason among others.

The system postulates that *Ishwara*, the spirit in man, is untouched by any troubles, works, fruit of works, or desires, and when a firm position is assumed with the end in view of reaching union with spirit through concentration, He comes to the aid of the lower self and raises it gradually to higher planes. In this process the Will by degrees is given a stronger and stronger tendency to act upon a different line from that indicated by passion and desire. Thus it is freed from the domination of desire and at last subdues the mind itself. But before the perfection of the practice is arrived at the will still acts according to desire, only that the desire is for higher things and away from those of the material life. Book III is for the purpose of defining the nature of the perfected state, which is therein denominated *Isolation.*

Isolation of the Soul in this philosophy does not mean that a man is isolated from his fellows, becoming cold and dead, but only that the Soul is isolated or freed from the bondage of matter and desire, being thereby able to act for the accomplishing of the aim of Nature and Soul, including all souls of all men. Such, in the Aphorisms, is clearly stated to be the purpose. It has become the habit of many superficial readers and thinkers, to say nothing of those who oppose the Hindu philosophy, to assert that Jivanmuktas or Adepts remove themselves from all life of men, from all activity, and any participation in human affairs, isolating themselves on inaccessible mountains where no human cry can reach their ears. Such a charge is directly contrary to the tenets of the philosophy which prescribes the method and means for reaching such a state. These Beings are certainly removed from human observation, but, as the philosophy clearly states, they have the whole of nature for their object, and this will include all living men. They may not appear to take any interest in transitory improvements or ameliorations, but they work behind the scenes of true enlightenment until such times as men shall be able to endure their appearance in mortal guise.

The term "knowledge" as used here has a greater meaning than we are accustomed to giving it. It implies full identification of the mind, for any length of time, with whatever object or subject it is directed to. Modern science and metaphysics do not admit that the mind can cognize outside of certain given methods and distances, and in most quarters the existence of soul is denied or ignored. It is held, for instance, that one cannot know the constituents and properties of a piece of stone without mechanical or chemical aids applied directly to the object; and that nothing can be known of the thoughts or feelings of another person unless they are expressed in words or acts. Where metaphysicians deal with soul they are vague and appear to be afraid of science, because it is not possible to analyze it and weigh its parts in a balance. Soul and Mind are reduced to the condition of limited instruments which take note of certain physical facts spread before them through mechanical aids. Or, in ethnological investigation, it is held that we can know such and such things about classes of men from observations made through sight, touch, sense of smell and hearing, in which case mind and soul are still mere recorders. But this system declares that the practicer who has reached certain stages, can direct his mind to a piece of stone, whether at a distance or nearby, or to a man or class of men, and by means of concentration, cognize all the inherent qualities of the objects as well as accidental peculiarities, and know all about the subject. Thus, in the instance of, say, one of the Easter Islanders, the ascetic will cognize not only that which is visible to the senses or to be known from long observation, or that has been recorded, but also deeply seated qualities, and the exact line of descent and evolution of the particular human specimen under examination. Modern science can know nothing of the Easter Islanders and only makes wild guesses as to what they are; nor can it with any certainty tell what is and from what came a nation so long before the eye of science as the Irish. In the ease of the Yoga practitioner he becomes, through the power of concentration, completely identified with the thing considered, and so in fact experiences in himself all the phenomena exhibited by the object as well as all its qualities.

To make it possible to admit all this, it is first required that the existence, use and function of an ethereal medium penetrating everywhere, called Astral Light or Akasa by the Hindus, should be admitted. The Universal distribution of this as a fact in nature is metaphysically expressed in the terms "Universal Brotherhood" and "Spiritual Identity." In it, through its aid, and by its use, the qualities and motions of all objects are universally cognizable. It is the surface, so to say, upon which all human actions and all things, thoughts and circumstances are fixed. The Easter Islander comes of a stock which has left its imprint in this Astral Light, and carries with him in indelible writing the history of his race. The ascetic in concentration fixes his attention upon this, and then reads the record lost to Science. Every thought of Herbert Spencer, Mill, Bain, or Huxley is fastened in the Astral Light together with the respective systems of Philosophy formulated by them, and all that the ascetic has to do is to obtain a single point of departure connected with either of these thinkers, and then to read in the Astral Light all that they have thought out. By Patanjali and his school, such feats as these relate to matter and not to spirit, although to Western ears they will sound either absurd, or if believed in, as relating to spirit.

In the things of the spirit and of the mind, the modern schools seem, to the sincere student of this Philosophy, to be woefully ignorant. What spirit may be is absolutely unknown, and indeed, it cannot yet be stated what it is not. Equally so with mental phenomena. As to the latter there is nothing but a medley of systems. No one knows what mind is. One says it is brain and another denies it; another declares it to be a function, which a fourth refuses to admit. As to memory, its place, nature and essential property, there is nothing offered but empiric deductions. To explain the simple fact of a man remembering a circumstance of his early youth, all that is said is, that it made an impression on his mind or brain, with no reasonable statement of what is the mind nor how or where the brain retains such vast quantities of impressions.

With such a chaos in modern psychological systems, the student of Patanjali feels justified in adopting something which will, at least, explain and embrace the greater number of facts, and it is to be found in the doctrines again brought forward by the Theosophical Society, relating to man as a Spirit; to a Spirit in nature: to the identity of all spiritual beings, and to all phenomena presented for our consideration.

WILLIAM Q. JUDGE.

New York, 1889.

Book 1. Concentration

1. Assuredly, the exposition of Yoga, or Concentration, is now to be made.[1]

2. Concentration, or Yoga, is the hindering of the modifications of the thinking principle.[2]

3. At the time of concentration the soul abides in the state of a spectator without a spectacle.[3]

4. At other times than that of concentration, the soul is in the same form as the modification of the mind.[4]

5. The modifications of the mind are of five kinds, and they are either painful or not painful;

6. They are, Correct Cognition, Misconception, Fancy, Sleep, and Memory.

7. Correct Cognition results from Perception, Inference, and Testimony.

8. Misconception is Erroneous Notion arising from lack of Correct

---

[1] The Sanskrit particle *atha*, which is translated "assuredly," intimates to the disciple that a distinct topic is to be expounded, demands his attention, and also serves as a benediction. Monier Williams says it is "an auspicious and inceptive participle often not easily expressed in English."

[2] In other words, the want of concentration of thought is due to the fact that the mind—here called "the thinking principle"—is subject to constant modifications by reason of its being diffused over a multiplicity of subjects. So "concentration" is equivalent to the correction of a tendency to diffuseness, and to the obtaining of what the Hindus call "one-pointedness," or the power to apply the mind, at any moment, to the consideration of a single point of thought, to the exclusion of all else.

Upon this Aphorism the method of the system hinges. The reason for the absence of concentration at any time is, that the mind is modified by every subject and object that comes before it; it is, as it were, transformed into that subject or object. The mind, therefore, is not the supreme or highest power; it is only a function, an instrument with which the soul works, feels sublunary things, and experiences. The brain, however, must not be confounded with the mind, for the brain is in its turn but an instrument for the mind. It therefore follows that the mind has a plane of its own, distinct from the soul and the brain, and what is to be learned is, to use the will, which is also a distinct power from the mind and brain, in such a way that instead of permitting the mind to turn from one subject or object to another just as they may move it, we shall apply it as a servant at any time and for as long a period as we wish, to the consideration of whatever we have decided upon.

[3] This has reference to the perfection of concentration, and is that condition in which, by the hindering of the modifications referred to in *Aphorism 2*, the soul is brought to a state of being wholly devoid of taint of, or impression by, any subject. The "soul" here referred to is not Atma, which is spirit.

[4] This has reference to the condition of the soul in ordinary life, when concentration is not practiced, and means that, when the internal organ, the mind, is through the senses affected or modified by the form of some object, the soul also—viewing the object through its organ, the mind—is, as it were, altered into that form; as a marble statue of snowy whiteness, if seen under a crimson light will seem to the beholder crimson and so is, to the visual organs, so long as that colored light shines upon it.

Cognition.

9. Fancy is a notion devoid of any real basis and following upon knowledge conveyed by words.[5]

10. Sleep is that modification of the mind which ensues upon the quitting of all objects by the mind, by reason of all the waking senses and faculties sinking into abeyance.

11. Memory is the not letting go of an object that one has been aware of.

12. The hindering of the modifications of the mind already referred to, is to be effected by means of Exercise and Dispassion.

13. Exercise is the uninterrupted, or repeated, effort that the mind shall remain in its unmoved state.[6]

14. This exercise is a firm position observed out of regard for the end in view, and perseveringly adhered to for a long time without intermission.[7]

15. Dispassion is the having overcome one's desires.[8]

16. Dispassion, carried to the utmost, is indifference regarding all else than soul, and this indifference arises from a knowledge of soul as distinguished from all else.

17. There is a meditation of the kind called "that in which there is distinct cognition," and which is of a four-fold character because of Argumentation, Deliberation, Beatitude, Egoism.[9]

---

[5] For instance, the terms "a hare's horns" and "the head of Rahu," neither of which has anything in nature corresponding to the notion. A person hearing the expression "the head of Rahu" naturally fancies that there is a Rahu who owns the head, whereas Rahu—a mythical monster who is said to cause eclipses by swallowing the sun—is all head and has no body; and, although the expression "a hare's horns" is frequently used, it is well known that there is no such thing in nature. Much in the same way people continue to speak of the sun's "rising" and "setting," although they hold to the opposite theory.

[6] This is to say that in order to acquire concentration we must, again and again, make efforts to obtain such control over the mind that we can, at any time when it seems necessary, so reduce it to an unmoved condition or apply it to any one point to the exclusion of all others.

[7] The student must not conclude from this that he can never acquire concentration unless he devotes every moment of his life to it, for the words "without intermission" apply but to the length of time that has been set apart for the practice.

[8] That is—the attainment of a state of being in which the consciousness is unaffected by passions, desires, and ambitions, which aid in causing modifications of the mind.

[9] The sort of meditation referred to is a pondering wherein the nature of that which is to be pondered upon is well known, without doubt or error, and it is a distinct cognition which excludes every other modification of the mind than that which is to be pondered upon.

1. The Argumentative division of this meditation is a pondering upon a subject with argument as to its nature in comparison with something else; as, for instance, the question whether mind is the product of matter or precedes matter.

2. The Deliberative division is a pondering in regard to whence have come, and where is the field of action, of the subtler senses and the mind.

3. The Beatific condition is that in which the higher powers of the mind, together

18. The meditation just described is preceded by the exercise of thought without argumentation. Another sort of meditation is in the shape of the self-reproduction of thought after the departure of all objects from the field of the mind.

19. The meditative state attained by those whose discrimination does not extend to pure spirit, depends upon the phenomenal world.

20. In the practice of those who are, or may be, able to discriminate as to pure spirit, their meditation is preceded by Faith, Energy, Intentness (upon a single point), and Discernment, or thorough discrimination of that which is to be known.[10]

21. The attainment of the state of abstract meditation is speedy, in the case of the hotly impetuous.

22. Because of the mild, the medium, and the transcendent nature of the methods adopted, there is a distinction to be made among those who practice Yoga.

23. The state of abstract meditation may be attained by profound devotedness toward the Supreme Spirit considered in its comprehensible manifestation as *Ishwara.*[11]

24. *Ishwara* is a spirit, untouched by troubles, works, fruits of works, or desires.

25. In *Ishwara* becomes infinite that omniscience which in man exists but as a germ.

26. Ishwara is the preceptor of all, even of the earliest of created beings, for He is not limited by time.

27. His name is OM.

28. The repetition of this name should be made with reflection upon its signification.[12]

---

with truth in the abstract, are pondered upon.

4. The Egoistic division is one in which the meditation has proceeded to such a height that all lower subjects and objects are lost sight of, and nothing remains but the cognition of the self, which then becomes a stepping-stone to higher degrees of meditation.

The result of reaching the fourth degree, called Egoism, is that a distinct recognition of the object or subject with which the meditation began is lost, and self-consciousness alone results; but this self-consciousness does not include the consciousness of the Absolute or Supreme Soul.

[10] It is remarked here by the commentator, that "in him who has Faith there arises Energy, or perseverance in meditation, and, thus persevering, the memory of past subjects springs up, and his mind becomes absorbed in Intentness, in consequence of the recollection of the subject, and he whose mind is absorbed in meditation arrives at a thorough discernment of the matter pondered upon."

[11] It is said that this profound devotedness is a preeminent means of attaining abstract meditation and its fruits. "*Ishwara*" is the Spirit in the body.

[12] Om is the first letter of the Sanskrit alphabet. Its utterance involves three sounds, those of long *au*, short *u*, and the "stoppage" or labial consonant *m*. To this tripartiteness is attached deep mystical symbolic meaning. It denotes, as distinct yet in union, *Brahma, Vishnu*, and *Siva*, or Creation, Preservation, and Destruction. As a whole, it implies "the Universe." In its application to man, *au* refers to the spark of Divine Spirit that is in

29. From this repetition and reflection on its significance, there come a knowledge of the Spirit and the absence of obstacles to the attainment of the end in view.

30. The obstacles in the way of him who desires to attain concentration are Sickness, Languor, Doubt, Carelessness, Laziness, Addiction to objects of sense, Erroneous Perception, Failure to attain any stage of abstraction, and Instability in any stage when attained.

31. These obstacles are accompanied by grief, distress, trembling, and sighing.

32. For the prevention of these, one truth should be dwelt upon.[13]

33. Through the practicing of Benevolence, Tenderness, Complacency, and Disregard for objects of happiness, grief, virtue, and vice, the mind becomes purified.[14]

34. Distractions may be combated by a regulated control or management of the breath in inspiration, retention, and exhalation.

35. A means of procurement of steadiness of the mind may be found in an immediate sensuous cognition;

36. Or, an immediate cognition of a spiritual subject being produced, this may also serve to the same end;

37. Or, the thought taking as its object someone devoid of passion—as, for instance, an ideally pure character—may find what will serve as a means;

38. Or, by dwelling on knowledge that presents itself in a dream, steadiness of mind may be procured;

39. Or, it may be effected by pondering upon anything that one approves.

40. The student whose mind is thus steadied obtains a mastery which extends from the Atomic to the Infinite.

41. The mind that has been so trained that the ordinary

---

humanity; *u*, to the body through which the Spirit manifests itself; and *m*, to the death of the body, or its resolvement to its material elements. With regard to the cycles affecting any planetary system, it implies the Spirit, represented by *au* as the basis of the manifested worlds; the body or manifested matter, represented by *u*, through which the spirit works; and represented by *m*, "the stoppage or return of sound to its source," the *Pralaya or Dissolution* of the worlds. In practical occultism, through this word reference is made to Sound, or Vibration, in all its properties and effects, this being one of the greatest powers of nature. In the use of this word as a practice, by means of the lungs and throat, a distinct effect is produced upon the human body. In *Aphorism 28* the name is used in its highest sense, which will necessarily include all the lower. All utterance of the word OM, as a practice, has a potential reference to the conscious separation of the soul from the body.

[13] Any accepted truth which one approves is here meant.

[14] The chief occasions for distraction of the mind are Covetousness and Aversion, and what the aphorism means is, not that virtue and vice should be viewed with indifference by the student, but that he should not fix his mind with pleasure upon happiness or virtue, nor with aversion upon grief or vice, in others, but should regard all with an equal mind; and the practice of Benevolence, Tenderness, and Complacency brings about cheerfulness of the mind, which tends to strength and steadiness.

modifications of its action are not present, but only those which occur upon the conscious taking up of an object for contemplation, is changed into the likeness of that which is pondered upon, and enters into full comprehension of the being thereof.

42. This change of the mind into the likeness of what is pondered upon, is technically called the Argumentative condition, when there is any mixing-up of the title of the thing, the significance and application of that title, and the abstract knowledge of the qualities and elements of the thing *per se.*

43. On the disappearance, from the plane of contemplation, of the title and significance of the object selected for meditation; when the abstract thing itself, free from distinction by designation, is presented to the mind only as an entity, that is what is called the Non-Argumentative condition of meditation.[15]

44. The Argumentative and Non-Argumentative conditions of the mind, described in the preceding two aphorisms, also obtain when the object selected for meditation is subtle, or of a higher nature than sensuous objects.

45. That meditation which has a subtle object in view ends with the indissoluble element called *primordial matter.*

46. The mental changes described in the foregoing, constitute "meditation with its seed."[16]

47. When Wisdom has been reached, through acquirement of the non-deliberative mental state, there is spiritual clearness.

48. In that case, then, there is that Knowledge which is absolutely free from Error.

49. This kind of knowledge differs from the knowledge due to testimony and inference; because, in the pursuit of knowledge based upon those, the mind has to consider many particulars and is not engaged with the general field of knowledge itself.

50. The train of self-reproductive thought resulting from this puts a stop to all other trains of thought.[17]

---

[15] These two aphorisms (42-43) describe the first and second stages of meditation, in the mind properly intent upon objects of a gross or material nature. The next aphorism has reference to the state when subtle, or higher, objects are selected for contemplative meditation.

[16] "Meditation with its seed" is that kind of meditation in which there is still present before the mind a distinct object to be meditated upon.

[17] It is held that there are two main trains of thought; (*a*) that which depends upon suggestion made either by the words of another, or by impression upon the senses or mind, or upon association; (*b*) that which depends altogether upon itself, and reproduces from itself the same thought as before. And when the second sort is attained, its effect is to act as an obstacle to all other trains of thought, for it is of such a nature that it repels or expels from the mind any other kind of thought. As shown in *Aphorism 48*, the mental state called "non-argumentative" is absolutely free from error, since it has nothing to do with testimony or inference, but is knowledge itself, and therefore from its inherent nature it puts a stop to all other trains of thought.

51. This train of thought itself, with but one object, may also be stopped, in which case "meditation without a seed" is attained.[18]

END OF THE FIRST BOOK.

---

[18] "Meditation without a seed" is that in which the brooding of the mind has been pushed to such a point that the object selected for meditation has disappeared from the mental plane, and there is no longer any recognition of it, but consequent progressive thought upon a higher plane.

Book 2. Means of Concentration

1. The practical part of Concentration is, Mortification, Muttering, and Resignation to the Supreme Soul.[19]

2. This practical part of concentration is for the purpose of establishing meditation and eliminating afflictions.

3. The afflictions which arise in the disciple are Ignorance, Egoism, Desire, Aversion, and a tenacious wish for existence upon the earth.

4. Ignorance is the field of origin of the others named, whether they be dormant, extenuated, intercepted, or simple.

5. Ignorance is the notion that the non-eternal, the impure, the evil, and that which is not soul are, severally, eternal, pure, good, and soul.

6. Egoism is the identifying of the power that sees with the power of seeing.[20]

7. Desire is the dwelling upon pleasure.

8. Aversion is the dwelling upon pain.

9. The tenacious wish for existence upon earth is inherent in all sentient beings, and continues through all incarnations, because it has self-reproductive power. It is felt as well by the wise as the unwise.[21]

10. The foregoing five afflictions, when subtle, are to be evaded by the production of an antagonistic mental state.

11. When these afflictions modify the mind by pressing themselves upon the attention, they are to be got rid of by meditation.

12. Such afflictions are the root of, and produce, results in both physical and mental actions or works, and they, being our merits or demerits, have their fruitage either in the visible state or in that which is unseen.

13. While that root of merit and demerit exists, there is a fructification during each succeeding life upon earth in rank, years,

---

[19] What is here meant by "mortification" is the practice laid down in other books, such as the *Dharma Shastra,* which includes penances and fastings; "muttering" is the semi-audible repetition of formulae also laid down, preceded by the mystic name of the Supreme Being given in *Aphorism 27, Book I*; "resignation to the Supreme Soul," is the consigning to the Divine, or the Supreme Soul, all one's works, without interest in their results.

[20] *i.e.* it is the confounding of the soul, which really sees, with the tool it uses to enable it to see, *viz.* the mind, or—to a still greater degree of error—with those organs of sense which are in turn the tools of the mind; as, for instance, when an uncultured person thinks that it is his eye which sees, when in fact it is his mind that uses the eye as a tool for seeing.

[21] There is in the spirit a natural tendency, throughout a Manvantara, to manifestation on the material plane, on and through which only, the spiritual monads can attain their development; and this tendency, acting through the physical basis common to all sentient beings, is extremely powerful and continues through all incarnations, helping to cause them, in fact, and re-producing itself in each incarnation.

pleasure, or pain.

14. Happiness or suffering results, as the fruit of merit and demerit, accordingly as the cause is virtue or vice.

15. But to that man who has attained to the perfection of spiritual cultivation, all mundane things are alike vexatious, since the modifications of the mind due to the natural qualities are adverse to the attainment of the highest condition; because, until that is reached, the occupation of any form of body is a hindrance, and anxiety and impressions of various kinds ceaselessly continue.

16. That which is to be shunned by the disciple is pain not yet come.[22]

17. From the fact that the soul is conjoined in the body with the organ of thought, and thus with the whole of nature, lack of discrimination follows, producing misconceptions of duties and responsibilities. This misconception leads to wrongful acts, which will inevitably bring about pain in the future.

18. The Universe, including the visible and the invisible, the essential nature of which is compounded of purity, action, and rest, and which consists of the elements and the organs of action, exists for the sake of the soul's experience and emancipation.

19. The divisions of the qualities are the diverse, the non-diverse, those which may be resolved once but no farther, and the irresolvable.[23]

20. The soul is the Perceiver; is assuredly vision itself pure and simple; unmodified; and looks directly upon ideas.

21. For the sake of the soul alone, the Universe exists.[24]

22. Although the Universe in its objective state has ceased to be, in respect to that man who has attained to the perfection of spiritual cultivation, it has not ceased in respect to all others, because it is common to others besides him.

23. The conjuncture of the soul with the organ of thought, and thus with nature, is the cause of its apprehension of the actual condition of the nature of the Universe and of the soul itself.

24. The cause of this conjuncture is what is to be quitted, and that cause is ignorance.

25. The quitting consists in the ceasing of the conjuncture, upon

---

[22] The past cannot be changed or amended; that which belongs to the experiences of the present cannot, and should not, be shunned; but alike to be shunned are disturbing anticipations or fears of the future, and every act or impulse that may cause present or future pain to ourselves or others.

[23] The "diverse" are such as the gross elements and the organs of sense; the "non-diverse," the subtle elements and the mind; the "once resolvable," the intellect, which can be resolved into undifferentiated matter but no farther; and the "irresolvable," indiscrete matter.

[24] The commentator adds: "Nature in energizing does not do so with a view to any purpose of her own, but with the design, as it were, expressed in the words 'let me bring about the soul's experience.'"

which ignorance disappears, and this is the Isolation of the soul.[25]

26. The means of quitting the state of bondage to matter is perfect discriminative knowledge, continuously maintained.[26]

27. This perfect discriminative knowledge possessed by the man who has attained to the perfection of spiritual cultivation, is of seven kinds, up to the limit of meditation.

28. Until this perfect discriminative knowledge is attained, there results from those practices which are conducive to concentration, an illumination more or less brilliant which is effective for the removal of impurity.

29. The practices which are conducive to concentration are eight in number: Forbearance, Religious Observances, Postures, Suppression of the breath, Restraint, Attention, Contemplation, and Meditation.

30. Forbearance consists in not killing, veracity, not stealing, continence, and not coveting.

31. These, without respect to rank, place, time, or compact, are the universal great duties.

32. Religious Observances are purification of both mind and body, contentment, austerity, inaudible mutterings, and persevering devotion to the Supreme Soul.

33. In order to exclude from the mind questionable things, the mental calling up of those things that are opposite is efficacious for their removal.

34. Questionable things, whether done, caused to be done, or approved of; whether resulting from covetousness, anger, or delusion; whether slight, or of intermediate character, or beyond measure; are productive of very many fruits in the shape of pain and ignorance; hence, the "calling up of those things that are opposite" is in every way advisable.

35. When harmlessness and kindness are fully developed in the Yogi [he who has attained to cultivated enlightenment of the soul], there is a complete absence of enmity, both in men and animals, among all that are near to him.

36. When veracity is complete, the Yogi becomes the focus for the Karma resulting from all works good or bad.

37. When abstinence from theft, in mind and act, is complete in the

---

[25] That which is meant in this and in the preceding two aphorisms is that the conjuncture of soul and body, through repeated reincarnations, is due to its absence of discriminative knowledge of the nature of the soul and its environment, and when this discriminative knowledge has been attained, the conjuncture, which was due to the absence of discrimination, ceases of its own accord.

[26] The import of this—among other things—is that the man who has attained to the perfection of spiritual cultivation maintains his consciousness, alike while in the body, at the moment of quitting it, and when he has passed into higher spheres; and likewise when returning continues it unbroken while quitting higher spheres, when re-entering his body, and in resuming action on the material plane.

Yogi, he has the power to obtain all material wealth.

38. When continence is complete, there is a gain of strength, in body and mind.[27]

39. When covetousness is eliminated, there comes to the Yogi a knowledge of everything relating to, or which has taken place in, former states of existence.[28]

40. From purification of the mind and body there arises in the Yogi a thorough discernment of the cause and nature of the body, whereupon he loses that regard which others have for the bodily form; and he also ceases to feel the desire of, or necessity for, association with his fellow-beings that is common among other men.

41. From purification of the mind and body also ensure to the Yogi a complete predominance of the quality of goodness, complacency, intentness, subjugation of the senses, and fitness for contemplation and comprehension of the soul as distinct from nature.

42. From contentment in its perfection the Yogi acquires superlative felicity.

43. When austerity is thoroughly practiced by the Yogi, the result thereof is a perfecting and heightening of the bodily senses by the removal of impurity.

44. Through inaudible muttering there is a meeting with one's favorite Deity.[29]

45. Perfection in meditation comes from persevering devotion to the Supreme Soul.

46. A posture assumed by a Yogi must be steady and pleasant.[30]

47. When command over the postures has been thoroughly attained, the effort to assume them is easy; and when the mind has become thoroughly identified with the boundlessness of space, the posture becomes steady and pleasant.

48. When this condition has been attained, the Yogi feels no

---

[27] It is not meant here that a student practicing continence solely, and neglecting the other practices enjoined, will gain strength. All parts of the system must be pursued concurrently, on the mental, moral, and physical planes.

[28] "Covetousness" here applies not only to coveting any object, but also to the desire for enjoyable conditions of mundane existence, or even for mundane existence itself.

[29] By properly uttered invocations—here referred to in the significant phrase "inaudible mutterings," the higher powers in nature, ordinarily unseen by man, are caused to reveal themselves to the sight of the Yogi; and inasmuch as all the powers in nature cannot be evoked at once, the mind must be directed to some particular force, or power in nature—hence the use of the term "with one's favorite Deity."

[30] For the clearing up of the mind of the student it is to be observed that the "postures" laid down in various systems of "Yoga" are not absolutely essential to the successful pursuit of the practice of concentration and attainment of its ultimate fruits. All such "postures," as prescribed by Hindu writers, are based upon an accurate knowledge of the physiological effects produced by them, but at the present day they are only possible for Hindus, who from their earliest years are accustomed to assuming them.

assaults from the pairs of opposites.[31]

49. Also, when this condition has been attained, there should succeed regulation of the breath, in exhalation, inhalation, and retention.

50. This regulation of the breath, which is in exhalation, inhalation, and retention, is further restricted by conditions of time, place, and number, each of which may be long or short.

51. There is a special variety of breath regulation which has reference to both that described in the last preceding aphorism and the inner sphere of breathing.[32]

52. By means of this regulation of the breath, the obscuration of the mind resulting from the influence of the body is removed.

53. And thus the mind becomes prepared for acts of attention.

54. Restraint is the accommodation of the senses to the nature of the mind, with an absence on the part of the senses of their sensibility to direct impression from objects.

55. Therefrom results a complete subjugation of the senses.

END OF THE SECOND BOOK.

---

[31] By "pairs of opposites" reference is made to the conjoined classification, all through the Hindu philosophical and metaphysical systems, of the opposed qualities, conditions, and states of being, which are eternal sources of pleasure or pain in mundane existence, such as cold and heat, hunger and satiety, day and night, poverty and riches, liberty and despotism.

[32] *Aphorisms 49, 50, 51* allude to regulation of the breath as a portion of the physical exercises referred to in the note upon *Aphorism 46*, acquaintance with the rules and prescriptions for which, on the part of the student, is inferred by Patanjali. *Aphorism 50* refers merely to the regulation of the several periods, degrees of force; and number of alternating recurrences of the three divisions of breathing—exhalation, inhalation, and retention of the breath. But *Aphorism 51* alludes to another regulation of the breath, which is its governance by the mind so as to control its direction to and consequent influence upon certain centers of nerve perception within the human body for the production of physiological, followed by psychic effects.

Book 3. The Doctrine of Salvation

1. Fixing the mind on a place, object, or subject is attention.[33]

2. The continuance of this attention is contemplation.[34]

3. This contemplation, when it is practiced only in respect to a material subject or object of sense, is meditation.[35]

4. When this fixedness of attention, contemplation, and meditation are practiced with respect to one object, they together constitute what is called *Sanyama.*[36]

5. By rendering *Sanyama*—or the operation of fixed attention, contemplation, and meditation—natural and easy, an accurate discerning power is developed.[37]

6. *Sanyama* is to be used in proceeding step by step in overcoming all modifications of the mind, from the more apparent to those the most subtle.[38]

7. The three practices—attention, contemplation, and meditation—are more efficacious for the attainment of that kind of meditation called, "that in which there is distinct cognition," than the first five means heretofore described as "not killing, veracity, not stealing, continence, and not coveting."[39]

8. Attention, contemplation, and meditation are anterior to and not immediately productive of that kind of meditation in which the distinct cognition of the object is lost, which is called meditation without a seed.

9. There are two trains of self-reproductive thought, the first of which results from the mind being modified and shifted by the object or subject contemplated; the second, when it is passing from that modification and is becoming engaged only with the truth itself; at the

---

[33] This is called *Dharana.*

[34] This is called *Dhyana.*

[35] This is called *Samádi.*

[36] We have no word in English corresponding to *Sanyama.* The translators have used the word *restraint,* but this is inadequate and misleading, although it is a correct translation. When a Hindu says that an ascetic is practicing restraint according to this system in respect to any object, he means that he is performing *Sanyama,* while in English it may indicate that he is restraining himself from some particular thing or act, and this is not the meaning of *Sanyama.* We have used the language of the text, but the idea may perhaps be better conveyed by "perfect concentration."

[37] This "discerning power" is a distinct faculty which this practice alone develops, and is not possessed by ordinary persons who have not pursued concentration.

[38] See note to *Aphorism 2, Book I.* The student is to know that after he has overcome the afflictions and obstructions described in the preceding books, there are other modifications of a recondite character suffered by the mind, which are to be got rid of by means of *Sanyama.* When he has reached that stage the difficulties will reveal themselves to him.

[39] See *Aphorism 17, Book I.*

moment when the first is subdued and the mind is just becoming intent, it. is concerned in both of those two trains of self-reproductive thought, and this state is technically called *Nirodha.*

10. In that state of meditation which has been called *Nirodha*, the mind has an uniform flow.

11. When the mind has overcome and fully controlled its natural inclination to consider diverse objects, and begins to become intent upon a single one, meditation is said to be reached.

12. When the mind, after becoming fixed upon a single object, has ceased to be concerned in any thought about the condition, qualities, or relations of the thing thought of, but is absolutely fastened upon the object itself, it is then said to be intent upon a single point—a state technically called *Ekagrata.*

13. The three major classes of perception regarding the characteristic property, distinctive mark or use, and possible changes of use or relation, of any object or organ of the body contemplated by the mind, have been sufficiently explained by the foregoing exposition of the manner in which the mind is modified.[40]

14. The properties of an object presented to the mind are: first, those which have been considered and dismissed from view; second, those under consideration; and third, that which is incapable of denomination because it is not special, but common to all matter.[41]

15. The alterations in the order of the three-fold mental modifications before described, indicate to the ascetic the variety of changes which a characteristic property is to undergo when contemplated.

16. A knowledge of past and future events comes to an ascetic from his performing *Sanyama* in respect to the three-fold mental modifications just explained.[42]

17. In the minds of those who have not attained to concentration, there is a confusion as to uttered sounds, terms, and knowledge, which results from comprehending these three indiscriminately; but when an ascetic views these separately, by performing "*Sanyama*" respecting them, he attains the power of understanding the meaning of any sound

---

[40] It is very difficult to put this aphorism into English. The three words translated as "characteristic property, distinctive mark or use, and possible change of use" are *Dharma*, *Lakshana*, and *Avastha*, and may be thus illustrated: *Dharma*, as, say, the clay of which a jar is composed, *Lakshana*, the idea of a jar thus constituted, and *Avastha*, the consideration that the jar alters every moment, in that it becomes old, or is otherwise affected.

[41] The third class above spoken of has reference to a tenet of the philosophy which holds that all objects may and will be finally "resolved into nature" or one basic substance; hence gold may be considered as mere matter, and therefore not different—not to be separately denominated in final analysis—from earth.

[42] See *Aphorism 4*, where "*Sanyama*" is explained as the use or operation of attention, contemplation, and meditation in respect to a single object.

uttered by any sentient being.

18. A knowledge of the occurrences experienced in former incarnations arises in the ascetic from holding before his mind the trains of self-reproductive thought and concentrating himself upon them.

19. The nature of the mind of another person becomes known to the ascetic when he concentrates his own mind upon that other person.

20. Such concentration will not, however, reveal to the ascetic the fundamental basis of the other person's mind, because he does not "perform *Sanyama*" with that object before him.

21. By performing concentration in regard to the properties and essential nature of form, especially that of the human body, the ascetic acquires the power of causing the disappearance of his corporeal frame from the sight of others, because thereby its property of being apprehended by the eye is checked, and that property of *Satwa* which exhibits itself as luminousness is disconnected from the spectator's organ of sight.[43]

22. In the same manner, by performing *Sanyama* in regard to any particular organ of sense—such as that of hearing, or of feeling, or of tasting, or of smelling—the ascetic acquires the power to cause cessation of the functions of any of the organs of another or of himself, at will.[44]

23. Action is of two kinds; first, that accompanied by anticipation of consequences; second, that which is without any anticipation of consequences. By performing concentration with regard to these kinds of action, a knowledge arises in the ascetic as to the time of his death.[45]

24. By performing concentration in regard to benevolence,

---

[43] Another great difference between this philosophy and modern science is here indicated. The schools of today lay down the rule that if there is a healthy eye in line with the rays of light reflected from an object—such as a human body—the latter will be seen, and that no action of the mind of the person looked at can inhibit the functions of the optic nerves and retina of the onlooker. But the ancient Hindus held that all things are seen by reason of that differentiation of *Satwa*—one of the three great qualities composing all things—which is manifested as luminousness, operating in conjunction with the eye, which is also a manifestation of *Satwa* in another aspect. The two must conjoin; the absence of luminousness or its being disconnected from the seer's eye will cause a disappearance. And as the quality of luminousness is completely under the control of the ascetic, he can, by the process laid down, check it, and thus cut off from the eye of the other an essential element in the seeing of any object.

[44] The ancient commentator differs from others with regard to this aphorism, in that he asserts that it is a portion of the original text, while they affirm that it is not, but an interpolation.

[45] *Karma*, resultant from actions of both kinds in present and in previous incarnations, produces and affects our present bodies, in which we are performing similar actions. The ascetic, by steadfastly contemplating all his actions in this and in previous incarnations (see *Aphorism 18*), is able to know absolutely the consequences resultant from actions he has performed, and hence has the power to calculate correctly the exact length of his life.

tenderness, complacency, and disinterestedness, the ascetic is able to acquire the friendship of whomsoever he may desire.

25. By performing concentration with regard to the powers of the elements, or of the animal kingdom, the ascetic is able to manifest those in himself.

26. By concentrating his mind upon minute, concealed or distant objects, in every department of nature, the ascetic acquires thorough knowledge concerning them.

27. By concentrating his mind upon the sun, a knowledge arises in the ascetic concerning all spheres between the earth and the sun.

28. By concentrating his mind upon the moon, there arises in the ascetic a knowledge of the fixed stars.

29. By concentrating his mind upon the polar star, the ascetic is able to know the fixed time and motion of every star in the *Brahmanda* of which this earth is a part.[46]

30. By concentrating his mind upon the solar plexus, the ascetic acquires a knowledge of the structure of the material body.

31. By concentrating his mind upon the nerve center in the pit of the throat, the ascetic is able to overcome hunger and thirst.

32. By concentrating his mind upon the nerve center below the pit of the throat, the ascetic is able to prevent his body being moved, without any resistant exertion of his muscles.

33. By concentrating his mind upon the light in the head the ascetic acquires the power of seeing divine beings.[47]

34. The ascetic can, after long practice, disregard the various aids to concentration hereinbefore recommended for the easier acquirement of knowledge, and will be able to possess any knowledge simply through the desire therefore.

35. By concentrating his mind upon the *Hridaya*, the ascetic acquires penetration and knowledge of the mental conditions, purposes, and thoughts of others, as well as an accurate comprehension of his own.[48]

---

[46] "*Brahmanda*" here means the great system, called by some "*universe*," in which this world is.

[47] There are two inferences here which have nothing to correspond to them in modern thought. One is, that there is a light in the head; and the other, that there are divine beings who may be seen by those who thus concentrate upon the "light in the head." It is held that a certain nerve, or psychic current, called *Brahmarandhra-nadi*, passes out through the brain near the top of the head. In this there collects more of the luminous principle in nature than elsewhere in the body and it is called *jyotis*—the light in the head. And, as every result is to be brought about by the use of appropriate means, the seeing of divine beings can be accomplished by concentration upon that part of the body more nearly connected with them. This point—the end of *Brahmarandhra-nadi*—is also the place where the connection is made between man and the solar forces.

[48] *Hridaya* is the heart. There is some disagreement among mystics as to whether the muscular heart is meant, or some nervous center to which it leads, as in the case of a similar direction for concentrating on the umbilicus, when, in fact, the field of nerves

36. By concentrating his mind upon the true nature of the soul as being entirely distinct from any experiences, and disconnected from all material things, and dissociated from the understanding, a knowledge of the true nature of the soul itself arises in the ascetic.

37. From the particular kind of concentration last described, there arises in the ascetic, and remains with him at all times, a knowledge concerning all things, whether they be those apprehended through the organs of the body or otherwise presented to his contemplation.

38. The powers hereinbefore described are liable to become obstacles in the way of perfect concentration, because of the possibility of wonder and pleasure flowing from their exercise, but are not obstacles for the ascetic who is perfect in the practice enjoined.[49]

39. The inner self of the ascetic may be transferred to any other body and there have complete control, because he has ceased to be mentally attached to objects of sense, and through his acquisition of the knowledge of the manner in and means by which the mind and body are connected.[50]

40. By concentrating his mind upon, and becoming master of, that vital energy called *Udana*, the ascetic acquires the power of arising from beneath water, earth, or other superincumbent matter.[51]

41. By concentrating his mind upon the vital energy called *Samana*, the ascetic acquires the power to appear as if blazing with light.[52]

42. By concentrating his mind upon the relations between the ear and *Akasa*, the ascetic acquires the power of hearing all sounds, whether upon the earth or in the ether, and whether far or near.[53]

43. By concentrating his mind upon the human body, in its relations to air and space, the ascetic is able to change at will the polarity of his body, and consequently acquires the power of freeing it

---

called the solar plexus is intended.

[49] "Practice enjoined," see *Aphorisms 36, 37.*

[50] As this philosophy holds that the mind, not being the result of brain, enters the body by a certain road and is connected with it in a particular manner, this aphorism declares that, when the ascetic acquires a knowledge of the exact process of connecting mind and body, he can connect his mind with any other body, and thus transfer the power to use the organs of the occupied frame in experiencing effects from the operations of the senses.

[51] *Udana* is the name given to one of the so-called "vital airs." These, in fact, are certain nervous functions for which our physiology has no name, and each one of which has its own office. It may be said that by knowing them, and how to govern them, one can alter his bodily polarity at will. The same remarks apply to the next aphorism.

[52] This effect has been seen by the interpreter on several occasions when in company with one who had acquired the power. The effect was as if the person had a luminousness under the skin.—W. Q. J.

[53] The word *Akasa* has been translated both as "ether" and "astral light." In this aphorism it is employed in the former sense. Sound, it will remembered, is the distinctive property of this element.

from the control of the laws of gravitation.

44. When the ascetic has completely mastered all the influences which the body has upon the inner man, and has laid aside all concern in regard to it, and in no respect is affected by it, the consequence is a removal of all obscurations of the intellect.

45. The ascetic acquires complete control over the elements by concentrating his mind upon the five classes of properties in the manifested universe; as, first, those of gross or phenomenal character; second, those of form; third, those of subtle quality; fourth, those susceptible of distinction as to light, action, and inertia; fifth, those having influence in their various degrees for the production of fruits through their effects upon the mind.

46. From the acquirement of such power over the elements there results to the ascetic various perfections, to wit, the power to project his inner-self into the smallest atom, to expand his inner-self to the size of the largest body, to render his material body light or heavy at will, to give indefinite extension to his astral body or its separate members, to exercise an irresistible will upon the minds of others, to obtain the highest excellence of the material body, and the ability to preserve such excellence when obtained.

47. Excellence of the material body consists in color, loveliness of form, strength, and density.

48. The ascetic acquires complete control over the organs of sense from having performed *Sanyama* (concentration) in regard to perception, the nature of the organs, egoism, the quality of the organs as being in action or at rest, and their power to produce merit or demerit from the connection of the mind with them.

49. Therefrom spring up in the ascetic the powers; to move his body from one place to another with the quickness of thought, to extend the operations of his senses beyond the trammels of place or the obstructions of matter, and to alter any natural object from one form to another.

50. In the ascetic who has acquired the accurate discriminative knowledge of the truth and of the nature of the soul, there arises a knowledge of all existences in their essential natures and a mastery over them.

51. In the ascetic who acquires an indifference even to the last mentioned perfection, through having destroyed the last germs of desire, there comes a state of the soul that is called Isolation.[54]

52. The ascetic ought not to form association with celestial beings who may appear before him, nor exhibit wonderment at their appearance, since the result would be a renewal of afflictions of the mind.

---

[54] See note on Isolation in Book IV.

53. A great and most subtle knowledge springs from the discrimination that follows upon concentration of the mind performed with regard to the relation between moments and their order.[55]

54. Therefrom results in the ascetic a power to discern subtle differences impossible to be known by other means.

55. The knowledge that springs from this perfection of discriminative power is called "knowledge that saves from rebirth." It has all things and the nature of all things for its objects, and perceives all that hath been and that is, without limitations of time, place, or circumstance, as if all were in the present and the presence of the contemplator.[56]

56. When the mind no longer conceives itself to be the knower, or experiencer, and has become one with the soul—the real knower and experiencer—Isolation takes place and the soul is emancipated.

END OF THE THIRD BOOK.

---

[55] In this Patanjali speaks of ultimate divisions of time which cannot be further divided, and of the order in which they precede and succeed each other. It is asserted that a perception of these minute periods can be acquired, and the result will be that he who discriminates thus goes on to greater and wider perception of principles in nature which are so recondite that modern philosophy does not even know of their existence. We know that we can all distinguish such periods as days or hours, and there are many persons, born mathematicians, who are able to perceive the succession of minutes and can tell exactly without a watch how many have elapsed between any two given points in time. The minutes, so perceived by these mathematical wonders, are, however, not the ultimate divisions of time referred to in the Aphorism, but are themselves composed of such ultimates. No rules can be given for such concentration as this, as it is so far on the road of progress that the ascetic finds the rules himself, after having mastered all the anterior processes.

[56] Such an ascetic as is referred to in this and the next aphorism, is a *Jivanmukta* and is not subject to reincarnation. He, however, may live yet upon earth but is not in any way subject to his body, the soul being perfectly free at every moment. And such is held to be the state of those beings called, in theosophical literature, Adepts, Mahatmas, Masters.

Book 4. The Essential Nature of Isolation

1. Perfections of body, or superhuman powers are produced by birth, or by powerful herbs, or by incantations, penances, or meditations.[57]

2. The change of a man into another class of being—such as that of a celestial being—is effected by the transfusion of natures.[58]

3. Certain merits, works, and practices are called "occasional" because they do not produce essential modification of nature; but they are effective for the removal of obstructions in the way of former merit, as in the case of the husbandman who removes impediments in the course of the irrigating stream, which then flows forward.[59]

4. The minds acting in the various bodies which the ascetic voluntarily assumes are the production of his egoism alone.

5. And for the different activities of those various minds, the ascetic's mind is the moving cause.

6. Among the minds differently constituted by reason of birth, herbs, incantations, penances, and meditation, that one alone which is due to meditation is destitute of the basis of mental deposits from works.[60]

7. The work of the ascetic is neither pure nor dark, but is peculiar to itself, while that of others is of three kinds.[61]

8. From these works there results, in every incarnation, a manifestation of only those mental deposits which can come to fructification in the environment provided.

9. Although the manifestation of mental deposits may be intercepted by unsuitable environments, differing as to class, place, and time, there is an immediate relation between them, because the memory

---

[57] The sole cause of permanent perfections is meditation performed in incarnations prior to that in which the perfection appears, for perfection by birth, such as the power of birds to fly, is impermanent, as also are those following upon incantations, elixirs and the like. But as meditation reaches within, it affects each incarnation. It must also follow that evil meditation will have the result of begetting perfection in evil.

[58] This alludes to the possibility—admitted by the Hindus—of a man's being altered into one of the *Devas*, or celestial beings, through the force of penances and meditation.

[59] This is intended to further explain *Aphorism 2* by showing, that in any incarnation certain practices (*e.g.* those previously laid down) will clear away the obscurations of a man's past *Karma*, upon which that *Karma* will manifest itself; whereas, if the practices were not pursued, the result of past meditation might be delayed until yet another life.

[60] The aphorism applies to all classes of men, and not to bodies assumed by the ascetic; and there must always be kept in view the doctrine of the philosophy that each life leaves in the Ego mental deposits which form the basis upon which subsequent vicissitudes follow in other lives.

[61] The three kinds of work alluded to are (1) pure in action and motive; (2) dark, such as that of infernal beings; (3) that of the general run of men, pure-dark. The 4th is that of the ascetic.

and the train of self-reproductive thought are identical.[62]

10. The mental deposits are eternal because of the force of the desire which produced them.[63]

11. As they are collected by cause, effect, substratum, and support, when those are removed, the result is that there is a non-existence of the mental deposits.[64]

12. That which is past and that which is to come, are not reduced to non-existence, for the relations of the properties differ one from the other.

13. Objects, whether subtle or not, are made up of the three qualities.[65]

14. Unity of things results from unity of modification.

15. Cognition is distinct from the object, for there is diversity of thoughts among observers of one object.

16. An object is cognized or not cognized by the mind accordingly as the mind is or is not tinted or affected by the object.

17. The modifications of the mind are always known to the presiding spirit, because it is not subject to modification.[66]

18. The mind is not self-illuminative, because it is an instrument of the soul, is colored and modified by experiences and objects, and is cognized by the soul.

19. Concentrated attention to two objects cannot take place simultaneously.

20. If one perception be cognizable by another, then there would be the further necessity for cognition of cognition, and from that a confusion of recollection would take place.

21. When the understanding and the soul are united, then self-

---

[62] This is to remove a doubt caused by *Aphorism 8*, and is intended to show that memory is not due to mere brain matter, but is possessed by the incarnating ego, which holds all the mental deposits in a latent state, each one becoming manifest whenever the suitable bodily constitution and environment are provided for it.

[63] In the Indian edition this reads that the deposits remain because of the "benediction." And as that word is used in a special sense, we do not give it here. All mental deposits result from a desire for enjoyment, whether it be from a wish to avoid in the next life certain pain suffered in this, or from the positive feeling expressed in the desire, "may such and such pleasure always be mine." This is called a "benediction." And the word "eternal" has also a special signification, meaning only that period embraced by a "day of Brahma," which lasts for a thousand ages.

[64] This aphorism supplements the preceding one, and intends to show that, although the deposits will remain during "eternity" if left to themselves—being always added to by new experiences and similar desires—yet they may be removed by removing producing causes.

[65] The "three qualities" are *Satwa*, *Rajas*, *Tamo*, or Truth, Activity, and Darkness: Truth corresponding to light and joy; Activity to passion; and Darkness to evil, rest, indifference, sloth, death. All manifested objects are compounded of these three.

[66] Hence, through all the changes to which the mind and soul are subject, the spiritual soul, *Ishwara*, remains unmoved, "the witness and spectator."

knowledge results.[67]

22. The mind, when united with the soul and fully conversant with knowledge, embraces universally all objects.

23. The mind, though assuming various forms by reason of innumerable mental deposits, exists for the purpose of the soul's emancipation and operates in co-operation therewith.

24. In him who knows the difference between the nature of soul and mind, the false notion regarding the soul comes to an end.[68]

25. Then the mind becomes deflected toward discrimination and bowed down before Isolation.

26. But in the intervals of meditation other thoughts arise, in consequence of the continuance of old impressions not yet expunged.

27. The means to be adopted for the avoidance and elimination of these are the same as before given for obviating the afflictions.

28. If the ascetic is not desirous of the fruits, even when perfect knowledge has been attained, and is not inactive, the meditation technically called *Dharma Megha*—cloud of virtue—takes place from his absolutely perfect discriminative knowledge.[69]

29. Therefrom results the removal of the afflictions and all works.

30. Then, from infinity of knowledge absolutely free from obscuration and impurity, that which is knowable appears small and easy to grasp.

31. Thereupon, the alternation in the modifications of the qualities, having accomplished the soul's aim—experience and emancipation—comes to an end.

32. It is then perceived that the moments and their order of precedence and succession are the same.[70]

---

[67] The self-knowledge spoken of here is that interior illumination desired by all mystics, and is not merely a knowledge of self in the ordinary sense.

[68] The mind is merely a tool, instrument, or means, by which the soul acquires experiences and knowledge. In each incarnation the mind is, as it were, new. It is a portion of the apparatus furnished to the soul through innumerable lives for obtaining experience and reaping the fruit of works performed. The notion that the mind is either knower or experiencer is a false one, which is to be removed before emancipation can be reached by soul. It was therefore said that the mind operates or exists for the carrying out of the soul's salvation, and not the soul for the mind's sake. When this is fully understood, the permanency of soul is seen, and all the evils flowing from false ideas begin to disappear.

[69] The commentator explains that, when the ascetic has reached the point described in *Aphorism 25*, if he bends his concentration toward the prevention of all other thoughts, and is not desirous of attaining the powers resulting just at his wish, a further state of meditation is reached which is called "cloud of virtue," because it is such as will, as it were, furnish the spiritual rain for the bringing about of the chief end of the soul—entire emancipation. And it contains a warning that, until that chief end is obtained, the desire for fruits is an obstacle.

[70] This is a step further than *Aphorism 53, Book III*, where it is stated that from discrimination of ultimates of time a perception of the very subtle and recondite principles of the universe results. Here, having arrived at *Isolation*, the ascetic sees

33. The reabsorption of the qualities which have consummated the aim of the soul or the abiding of the soul united with understanding in its own nature, is Isolation.[71]

END OF THE FOURTH BOOK

May Ishwara be near and help those who read this book.

OM

---

beyond even the ultimates, and they, although capable of affecting the man who has not reached this stage, are for the ascetic identical, because he is a master of them. It is extremely difficult to interpret this aphorism; and in the original it reads that "*the order is counterpart of the moment*." To express it in another way, it may be said that in the species of meditation adverted to in *Aphorism 53, Book III*, a calculative cognition goes forward in the mind, during which, the contemplator not yet being thoroughly master of these divisions of time, is compelled to observe them as they pass before him.

[71] This is a general statement of the nature of Isolation, sometimes called Emancipation. The qualities before spoken of, found in all objects and which had hitherto affected and delayed the soul, have ceased to be mistaken by it for realities, and the consequence is that the soul abides in its own nature unaffected by the great "pairs of opposites"—pleasure and pain, good and evil, cold and heat, and so forth.

Yet it must not be deduced that the philosophy results in a negation, or in a coldness, such as our English word "Isolation" would seem to imply. The contrary is the case. Until this state is reached, the soul, continually affected and deflected by objects, senses, suffering, and pleasure, is unable to consciously partake universally of the great life of the universe. To do so, it must stand firmly "in its own nature"; and then it proceeds further—as is admitted by the philosophy—to bring about the aim of all other souls still struggling on the road. But manifestly further aphorisms upon that would be out of place, as well as being such as could not be understood, to say nothing of the uselessness of giving them.